10 MIN

BEAUTY HACKS

SLEEP IN, SAVE MONEY, AND LOOK GREAT

DRAGON FRUIT

MARIA LLORENS

DISCLAIMER

Managing your beauty routine can be complicated, but we've broken down the best and worst of it to make it as easy as can be. From fixing a broken nail to de-puffing your eyes, we've got the hacks you need to look good and get out the door in no time at all. Our hacks don't shy away from the nitty gritty of all the beauty products, eye shadow techniques, contouring, and everything else you need to look good fast.

If you're confused about what to do with your face, hair, and nails—this guide is for you. We've tried to get all the best and most practical hacks in one book to make sure you look good in just a couple of minutes. We can't make you look like a celebrity or some other nonsense, but we can help you look like the best version of you.

"To start telling people that you're beautiful, or just feel beautiful, just start acting like you are the most beautiful woman in the world."

— Margaret Cho

CONTENTS

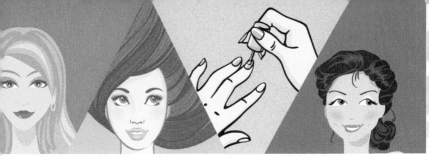

CHAPTER 5 // Complete Morning Looks   85

PREFACE

You're beautiful, grrrl. Or guy. Or they. Whatever your identification as a human being, we want you to feel your best every morning of your wonderful life. While there are many ways to accomplish this, we're going to focus on the more glamorous option — make up!

Make up shouldn't be a chore, and it's not even a requirement. It should always be a fun little tool in your arsenal of things that make you look fantastic. With our hacks, we'll answer all the finer points of how to get your beauty routine from boring drudgery to streamlined fun. How do you look more awake in the morning? How do you fix a broken nail or an old manicure? We've got a hack for all of your beauty problems.

So sit back, pull out your make up box, and let's learn a thing or two about making your morning routine simple and stress-free.

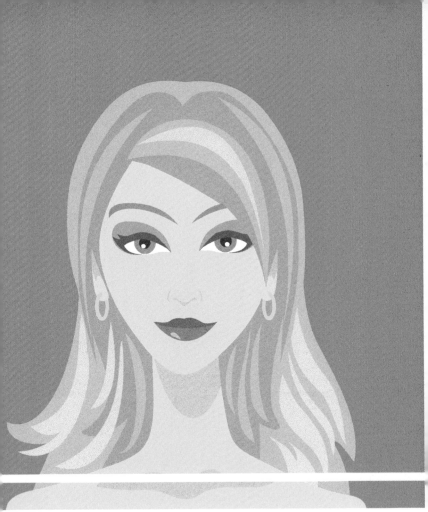

CHAPTER 1 //
Face and Lips

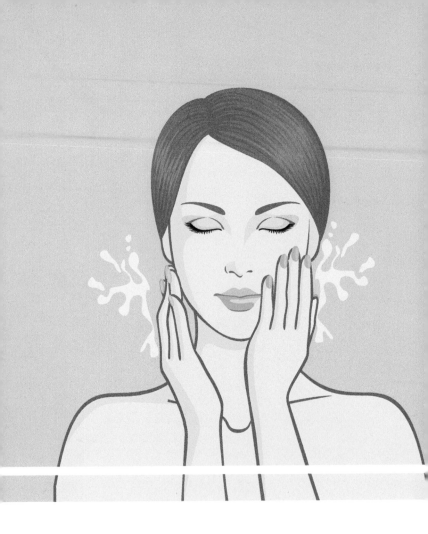

Face and Lips //
Morning Skin

W e all wake up sometimes feeling like we'd rather go back to sleep—or even like we just got hit by a train. On mornings like that, it's pretty unlikely we'd even want to put on make-up. That's why we've rounded up the best skin tricks to get your skin looking and feeling great. You don't have to sit for an hour with cucumbers on your eyes.

Hack 1: Hydrate While You Sleep

Don't waste time in the morning with moisturizer. Your skin will look even better if you pick a good moisturizer and let it sit overnight while you sleep.

Tip! It's better to apply to damp skin after you shower. And don't forget to moisturize your neck!

Hack 2: Multitask on Your Skin

You can save time on lathering up with lotion by using a hydrating exfoliating body wash in the shower.

Hack 3: Sleep with a Humidifier

Sleeping with a humidifier will help hydrate your skin overnight. Your skin will be less dry, itchy, and more supple. This is especially true in the winter, and it'll cut time off your morning routine.

Hack 4: Spot Treatment for Acne

Before bed, use a spot acne treatment containing a combination of sulfur and salicylic acid. After cleaning your face, use a Q-tip to apply a spot treatment directly to any new blemishes.

Hack 5: Soothe Irritation

Use a loose mineral powder with titanium dioxide or zinc oxide to reduce redness on your face. Dust with these and you'll get anti-inflammatory benefits that won't clog your pores.

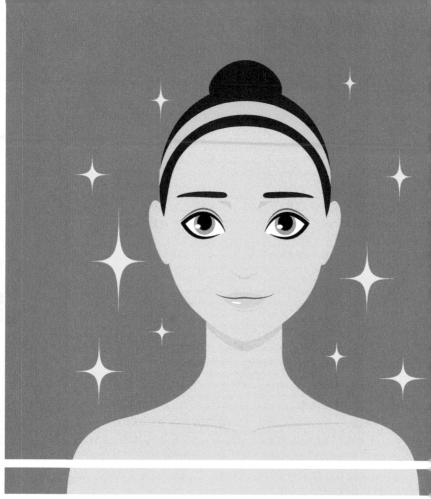

Face and Lips //
Looking Awake

Your eyes are one of the main attractions on your face, but they sometimes don't cooperate in the morning. You want to just get out the door but you look like you haven't slept and maybe like you've put on a few years in the past few hours. Let's look into how we can enhance the skin around your eyes.

Hack 1: De-puff Your Eyes Fast

There are plenty of cheap remedies to place on your eyes in the morning—cucumber slices, tea bags, frozen vegetables, cold spoons, etc. — but if you don't have time for any of those in the morning, then head to the store and get a roll-on eye product. Get rid of those puffy bags.

Hack 2: Exfoliate

Washing with an exfoliating scrub will create friction on your skin and increase blood flow, making it look brighter and more awake. Get rid of dead skin and get that pretty glow.

Tip! Rinse with cool water to reduce swelling.

Hack 3: Protect Your Skin

Double up on the skin treatment with a moisturizer that also has sunblock in it. You'll refresh and protect your skin at the same time.

Hack 4: 1-Minute Massage

You typically don't think of giving your skin a massage, but it's possible! Buy some oil specifically made for your face, and rub the oil gently into your face, wiping off any excess oil afterward.

Hack 5: Line Your Eyes

Using a nude or light-colored eyeliner will make your eyes look more awake, by making them look bigger. And use a smidge of highlighting eye shadow in the corners to increase the effect.

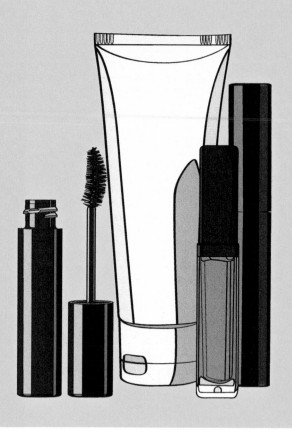

Face and Lips //
One Product Makeover

You have so many make up products, but you wish just one would magically transform your face into something present-able every rushed morning. It's a tough proposition, but we have a few tricks for when you really have no time at all.

Hack 1: Tinted Moisturizer with Sunscreen

Grab 'n' go with your tinted moisturizer. Your face will look fresh and will be protected with that good ol' SPF. Don't worry about perfection, a sheer formula is easy to apply even without a mirror.

Hack 2: Cream Blush

The easiest make up product you'll ever use. Look for a sheer formula in a neutral shade, like a bronze, and you can use it on your eyelids, too. If you have time, pair it with the tinted moisturizer for an extra polished finish.

Hack 3: Soft Eyeliner Pencil

Don't bother struggling in the morning with scraping your eyelid with a hard pencil—it's hard to apply and blend. Look for a soft pencil for automatic blending and quicker applica-tion. And it'll look less harsh for your morning look.

Hack 4: Mascara

Mascara makes a major impact to open up your eyes, so if there's only one thing you can put on in the morning, it's a good choice—especially if you have light-colored lashes. Choose a no-clump formula and don't even spend 30 sec-onds on this one.

Hack 5: Red Lipstick

You'll always look chic with red lipstick, so if it's all you can manage to get on in the morning, go for it. It may seem like a little much, but go for a lighter shade and your lips will look plump and flushed.

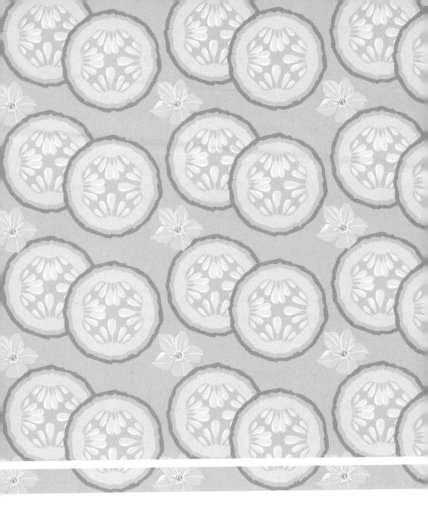

**Face and Lips //
Cheat Sleep**

If you really went all out the night before and didn't get any sleep, you're going to need something more than the hacks we suggested above. Let's get into some great under-eye tricks and a few natural remedies to make it easier to erase your lack of rest.

Hack 1: Red Lipstick and Concealer

It sounds weird, but it works! Use an orangey-red lipstick and apply with a brush all around the under-eye area before applying concealer. You'll get a much better result and get rid of those dark circles.

Hack 2: Q-Tips and Lashes

Boost your lashes with translucent powder and Q-tips! Apply one coat of mascara, then run the Q-tip along your lashes before the next coat of mascara. They'll appear more voluminous, which makes you look more awake.

Tip! Focus on the inner lashes for an even better effect.

Hack 3: Cucumber Cool

Put cucumbers in a bowl of cold water, and let them soak in there for a while. Then, submerge your face in the bowl (We know, it's so cold!) for as long as you can and then dry your face. Because of high antioxidant levels, cucumbers supposedly help fight aging and liven up your skin.

Hack 4: Use Spoons

Take two spoons from the kitchen and put them in the freezer to cool. While you make breakfast or coffee, let them get chilly for 10-20 minutes. Remove them from the freezer and gently press them (curve side down) onto your eyes. Holding them here for a few minutes will help de-puff and soothe tired eyes.

Hack 5: Strawberry Brightener

An alternate version of the cucumber trick, but try it with strawberries. Fresh strawberries are rich in vital nutrients, vitamins, minerals and rank among the top ten fruits and vegetables in terms of antioxidant capacity, making them perfect for boosting skin. Strawberries contain salicyl-ic acid, which helps remove dead cells and impurities while tightening pores. The fruit also has skin-lightening properties and is a traditional treatment for removing age spots and freckles.

Hack 6: Triangle Concealer

Apply a thin layer of concealer under the eye at the in-ner corner and extend downward to the cheek in the shape of a triangle (not a half moon). This shape works to brighten your under eye area and is less likely to be-come cakey in the corners of your eyes. Don't forget to blend well.

Hack 7: Circulate with Tea

Tea has great anti-inflammatory properties and it con-tains caffeine, beta-carotene, and vitamin C—all ex-tracts that improve circulation, tone, and structure of your skin. Drink tea in the morning to get these great effects on your skin.

Hack 8: Oatmeal Scrub

Take one tablespoon of oatmeal and add a bit of warm water (3 tablespoons or more) and wait a few minutes until oats become soft. Gently in a circular motion, mas-sage your clean face with this scrub to exfoliate your skin. Avoid the eye area since it's too rough. Rinse with warm water, then cold water. Oatmeal has anti-inflammatory and antioxidant properties, making it an ideal alternative to traditional face scrub. You can have it for breakfast and remove dead skin cells in the same morning!

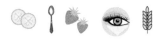

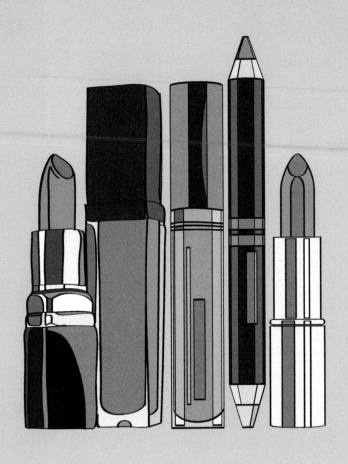

Face and Lips //
Luscious Lips

Your lips define the lower part of your face, so don't forget about their potential. There are plenty of ways to easily care for them and make them look good. Whether you just want to moisturize and perfect them or give your lips a bright, bold color, we've got just the thing.

Hack 1: Mascara Wand Exfoliator

For smoother lipstick application on dry lips, exfoliate with a clean and disposable mascara wand you may have lying around. Apply a lip balm over your mouth first so it's easier for the wand to get the dead skin off.

Hack 2: No-Rouge Teeth

Keep lipstick off your teeth by sticking your clean index finger in your mouth. Wrap your lips around it and pull it out. Any lipstick that would have gotten on your teeth is now on your finger. Crisis avoided!

Hack 3: Eye Shadow Re-use

If your favorite shadow crumbles and it's a color you'd also wear on your lips, store the broken pieces in a tiny container and mix what's left with some balm on a spoon, and then apply.

Hack 4: Long-Lasting Lipstick

You can make any lipstick last longer on your lips with translucent powder. First, put on your lip color and hold a tissue over your mouth. With the tissue on your mouth, dust your lips with translucent powder. A small amount will transfer this way, locking in your lipstick for all-day wear.

Hack 5: Perfect Color

To ensure that your lips will look like the color on your lipstick's packaging, use a small amount of concealer over them before you apply the lipstick. If your lips have a lot of pink or red in them, they'll benefit from this hack.

Hack 6: Bigger Lips

Another trick with concealer involves making your lips look larger. Cover your lips with concealer, then trace slightly outside your natural lip line with a lip liner pencil. You'll make them look larger that way.

Hack 7: 'X' Marks the Spot

For a perfect Cupid's bow lip, draw an 'X' on the center of your upper lip. Fully line and fill the rest of your lips. Don't just line the 'X' since it'll be very noticeable when your lipstick starts to wear off.

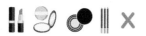

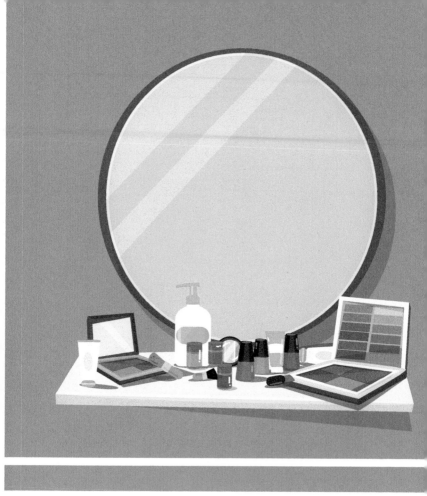

Face and Lips //
De-Clutter Your Products

You've got a bag full of make up, but you only use maybe half of it. It's time to ditch some of your products in order to clean up your routine. Not knowing what products to use every day is slowing you down and making it harder to get out the door fast.

Hack 1: Multitasking Products

Invest in some multitasking products. Save time by using brown eyeliner pencil to line your lashes, color your lids, and fill in your brows. And tint your cheeks and lips with a two-in-one stain. And make sure your moisturizers have SPF in them.

Hack 2: Expiration Dates

If it's more than a year old, chuck it. You don't want to use a product that's expired—especially sunscreen. Certain ingredients can cause unwanted reactions when they're expired.

Tip! Write down the purchase dates of all of your products on the bottom of the bottle.

Hack 3: Think Seasonal

You only need certain products during certain seasons, like a super-exfoliator. Those are useful during the winter, but less necessary in the summer when there's usually less dryness. Use it up and then toss it out, and make more room for stuff you really need—like moisturizer.

Hack 4: Say Goodbye

A general rule of thumb for de-cluttering is: if you wouldn't notice it's gone, get rid of it. Chances are you gravitate toward one or two of any particular category of make up—you have two favorite lipstick shades, for instance. If so, get the other products out of your main make up bag and give them away or toss them out. Chances are they may even be expired.

Hack 5: Donate

When you're throwing things out, try to donate before heading straight to the trash. Many women's shelters will take new and gently used products for the women they serve. Call your local shelter and ask what they accept. Other organizations accept make up for women as well.

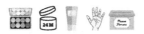

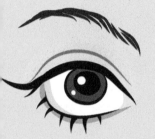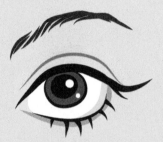

**CHAPTER 2 //
EYES**

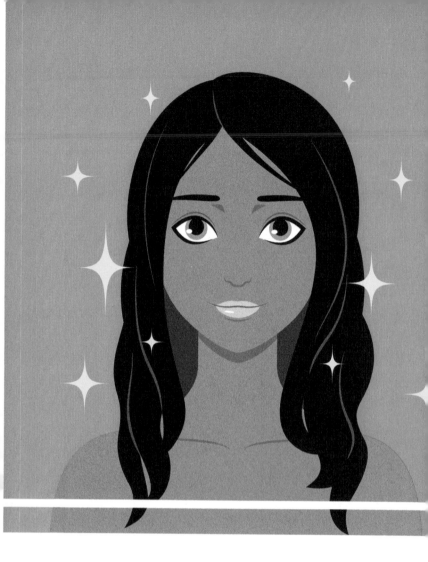

Eyes //
Simple Eye Looks

Eye makeup can be a difficult thing to master, even for beauty buffs. Sometimes it's easier to simplify in the morning rather than going for the most elaborate look. Here are a few of our favorite tricks for getting your eyes up to shape in no time at all.

Hack 1: Skip the Mascara

Applying mascara can often be messy, especially if you're in a rush. Swipe some Vaseline on your lashes instead of mascara to avoid a mess. Use a clean spoolie brush, roll it in Vaseline, and apply it to your lashes as you would mascara. You can also carefully use your fingertips if you're out of brushes. Not only will your lashes look longer and thicker, Vaseline helps moisturize them and encourages growth.

Hack 2: Skip Liquid Liner

Nobody has time to mess with crooked liquid lines in the morning. Stick to products that require less hassle in the morning, like pencil liner—which gives you the perfect line without the smudges. No need for damage control. You can also get the look of liquid liner with a good, soft kohl pencil which swipes on fast with no fuss and lasts all day.

Hack 3: Bright and Bold

Like the lipstick rule, if you go with a bright and bold color on your eyes, you won't need much else. Try a bright blue liner, swipe on some lip gloss, and you're all set. And remember to use white eye shadow as a base for extra pop.

Hack 4: Crease-Free Eyes

Concealer can crease if you have a few wrinkles, even if it is great for hiding under eye circles. Apply a light primer to your under eye area before adding concealer. And remember to use a beauty blending sponge and dab softly for fewer lines. Add powder for a smooth finish and no creases.

Hack 5: Apply Like a Pro

Getting the natural look with your eye makeup can seem difficult. Apply liquid or gel eyeliner before you apply your shadow to make it easier. Don't go overboard with eyeliner—it should be subtle for the natural look. When applying shadow, remember to keep dark shadow closest to the lashes, medium on top of that, and then the lightest toward the top of the eyelid.

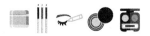

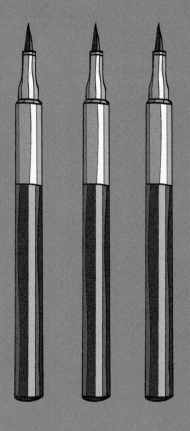

Eyes //
Perfect Lines

So you want a more polished look? Never fear, there are lots of ways to get those eyeliner lines looking smooth and shapely without a huge mess and a ton of time.

Hack 1: Purrfect Cat Eye

If drawing a cat eye is like painting Renaissance-quality portraits on your eyelids, save yourself time and pain by making a stencil. On a small piece of paper, cut your desired cat-eye shape and hold it up to your eyelids as you apply your liner. Even easier? Use a straight edge like a spoon or a credit card to outline the perfect shape every time.

Hack 2: Line and Curl

If you're really pressed for time, you can line your eyes and curl your lashes in one step. Draw a line using either a eyeliner pencil or gel liner (avoid liquid liner because it smudges too easily) across the edge of your eyelash curler where it would be touching your lid right above your lashes, curl, and out you go! Instantly lined lids and curled lashes.

Hack 3: Heat It Up

A pencil eyeliner becomes gel-like when you heat it up with a match or lighter. This means faster application for you. Hold your eye pencil in any color under the flame for one second, let it cool for 15 seconds, and then watch the consistency change right before your eyes. Finally, glide on your newly made gel liner for an instantly smoother formula.

Hack 4: Mascara Liner

If you've run out of eyeliner, use mascara instead to line your eyes in a pinch. Simply use a liner brush to collect the pigment off of the mascara brush, and use it to line your upper eyelid.

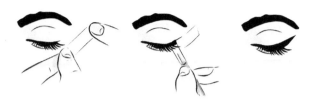

Hack 5: Scotch Tape Eyeliner

To get a nice curve with your eyeliner shape, take an inch-long piece of Scotch tape and press it onto your hand a few times to make it less sticky. This will make it less harsh on the delicate skin of your eye area. Place the tape underneath your bottom lashes at the outer corner of your eye and angle it toward your temple. With the tape guiding you, line as usual and draw a stripe to the outer corner of your eye and then out onto the tape. Remove tape, and voila!

Tip! Make sure the liner gets thinner and thinner as you sketch out the line.

How to : **CAT EYE**

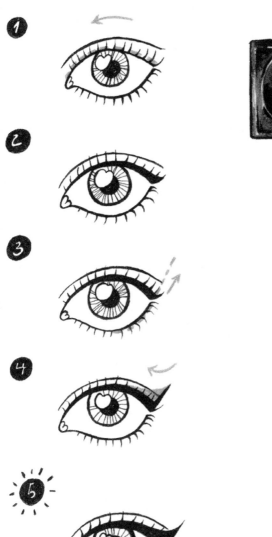

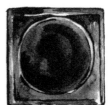

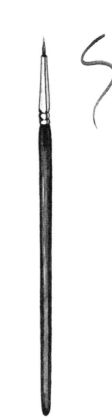

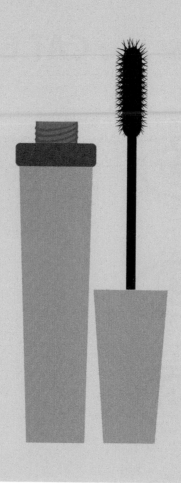

Eyes //
Better Lashes

Here are lots of ways to make your lashes look better than to simply pile on the mascara. And they'll probably make less of a mess and be less itchy when a bit of mascara globs into your eye. Here are our favorite hacks for pretty, long lashes.

Hack 1: Avoid Mascara Clumps

To avoid getting mascara clumps on your lashes, which would require extra cleanup time, roll your mascara brush over a tissue before applying. Make sure to only do it once, or you might remove too much formula from the mascara and waste some of that precious black gunk.

Hack 2: The Business Card Trick

Don't bother messing around trying to figure out your mascara in the morning. Get flawless lashes every morning with this do-ahead business card trick.

Just hold a business card above your eye, and using a pencil or pen, measure and mark the length of your eye, then connect the two marks by drawing the curve of your eye (it doesn't have to be perfect). Cut out that semicircle from the business card. Now place the cutout card over your eye, behind your lashes, and lift a little. Your lashes should lift up with your lid. Apply mascara as usual. Your messy mistakes will go on the card instead of your skin!

Hack 3: Saline Solution

Get your mascara running again with saline solution (the kind you use for your eyes). It will re-wet the flaky mascara. Remember, though, you're only supposed to keep mascara for three months. Any longer and it can lead to bacteria and eye infections. However, if it dries up within that time, revive it with this trick.

Hack 4: Hair Dryer Lashes

Hit your eyelash curler with a hair dryer to heat it up, so your lashes curl more easily. Blowing hot air on your eyelash curler will help your lashes curl easier and stay curled longer. It works the same way as if you were changing the texture of your hair with a hair iron or blow dryer. To do it, hit the lash curler with your blow dryer until it heats up, wait until it cools slightly but is still warm (don't burn yourself!), and then clamp down on your lashes to curl them.

Hack 5: Bobby Eyelash

A bobby pin has a lot of great uses, but did you know it's great for applying false lashes? Simply apply eyelash glue to the falsies with a clean bobby pin. Disperse the glue even along the base of the lashes. Wait a bit for the glue to get tacky and then apply.

Hack 6: The Bra Trick

To get the most out of your mascara, stick it in your bra for a few minutes to warm it up. It'll curl your lashes a lot better.

Hack 7: Baby Powder Lashes

Baby powder has a lot of great uses, like replacing dry shampoo, but it can also get you fuller, longer lashes. Simply dip a cotton swab into baby powder and run it across your lashes after your first coat of mascara. Then apply a second coat. The powder will adhere to the mascara, giving your lashes a great, almost-false lash look.

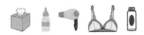

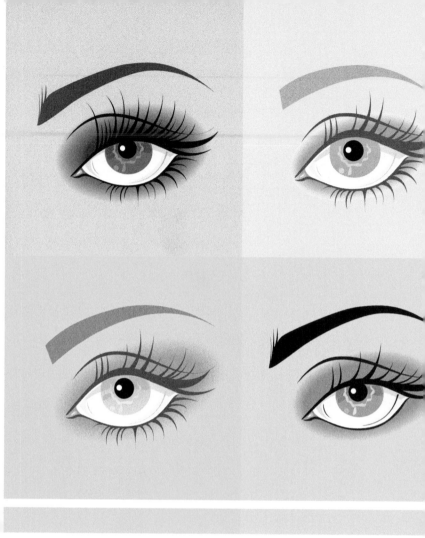

Eyes //
Eye Shadow Tricks

Sometimes eye shadow application can feel like smudging a bunch of product on your eyelid and hoping for the best. Don't settle for that mess, use some of these tricks to get the best smoky or brightly colored lids you're dreaming of.

Hack 1: White Eyelids

Ever wanted a matte, bright eye shadow look? Simply apply white liner to make sheer or less pigmented eye shadow appear more colorful than it is. Take a white eyeliner pencil and run it over the entire eyelid. The white base of the liner will intensify any eye shadow shade and make it pop instantly against your skin for a brighter, bolder look.

Hack 2: Hashtag Shadow

Draw a slanted hashtag at the outer corner of your eye, and then blend it for an instantly smoky effect. To create a super-easy smoky eye, draw a hashtag symbol right before the outer corner of your eye and then blend it out with the smudger at the other end of your eye liner.

Hack 3: Clean Smokey Eyes

It is important that you use one brush to apply your chosen colors and a clean brush to blend, especially if you're going for a smoky eye look. This keeps the colors from running into each other, particularly on your second eye when you have additional makeup on the brush. Clean your brush when you are finished so that it will be ready for tomorrow's morning rush.

Hack 4: Simple Intense Eyes

First, apply foundation or an eye shadow base on your eyelid. Then, apply a light color, like white or silver, in the inner corner of your eye. Apply a darker color on the outer corner, and blend the two in the middle. Apply black or your darkest color in your scheme to the outermost corner. Then line your upper and lower eyelids. Apply mascara and you're done!

Hack 5: Pencil-Only Eye Shadow

First, line your upper lash line then draw another line directly above that one. Keep drawing lines above each other until you reach your eye crease. Blend back and forth with a blending brush (or your finger if you don't have one), but don't go past where your eyebrows end.

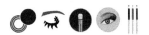

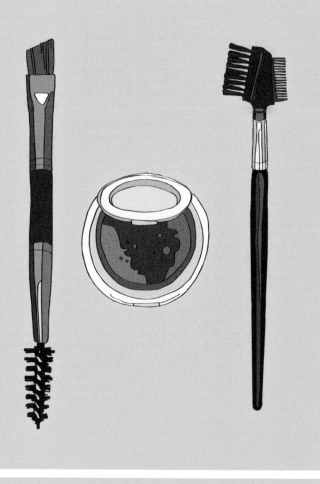

Eyes //
Excellent Eyebrows

Your brows frame your face, so don't forget about them. Whether you want a fuller look or simply to clean them up, your brows can be easy to pretty up. Simply follow these tips and you'll get the sharp, thick eyebrows you want.

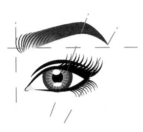

Hack 1: Find Your Arch

First, use a brush or a pencil to see where your eyebrows should start and end, and where the arch should go. Line up the brush with the corner of your eye diagonally to see where it ends, and with the inner corner of your eyelid to see where it begins. Then line it up with the outside of your pupil diagonally to see where your arch goes.

Hack 2: Fill 'Em In

You can fill in your brows with a pencil or powder and an angled brush—use whichever one you're most comfortable with. If your brows are particularly sparse, we suggest two-step approach. Use a powder to create the shape and then with a very thin pencil, use wispy light feathery strokes to create the illusion of real hairs.

Tip! Use a spoolie brush to brush out the pigment.

Hack 3: Brows That Pop

To make your brows pop, use a white liner or shadow to highlight the tops and bottoms. Then blend with a brush!

Hack 4: No Make Up Brows

Even if you're not a big fan of wearing makeup, you can still groom your brows and make 'em look fierce by brushing, trimming, and tweezing your eyebrows.

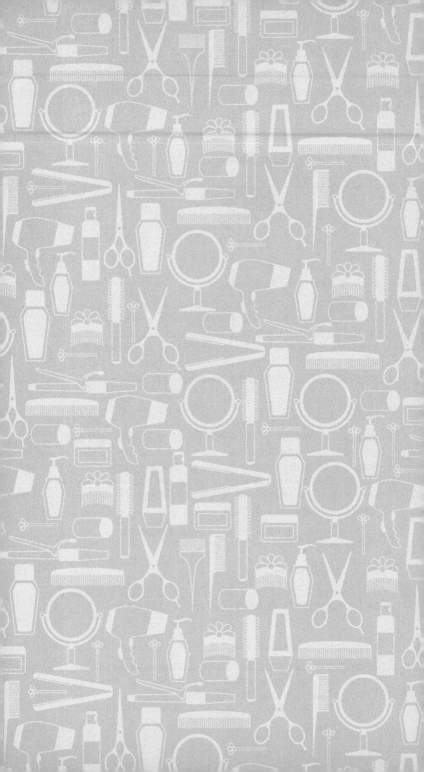

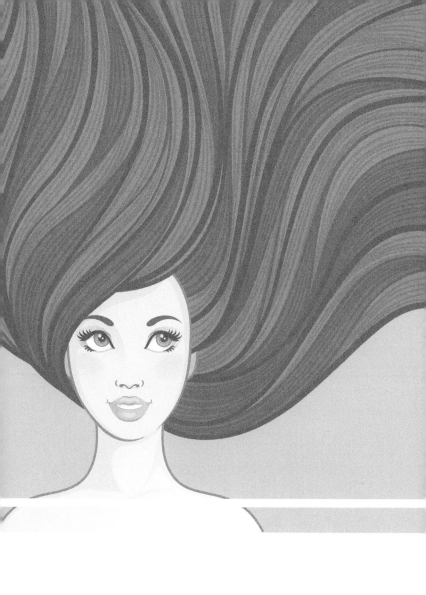

CHAPTER 3 //
Hair

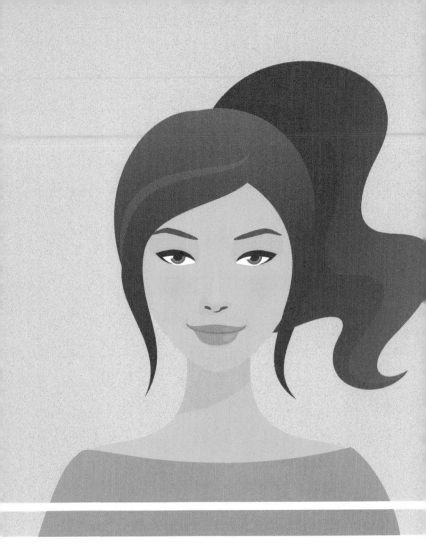

Hair //
Quick Morning Hair

Ugh! With tangles, dirty hair, and flatness, it's a miracle you ever wear anything other than a ponytail in the morning. Here are a few ways to upgrade from your everyday style for fast, chic looks.

Hack 1: Style the Night Before

Prep the night before to get the gorgeous waves that you want, even if you wake up with only enough time to throw on clothes and walk out the door. Before you go to bed, work texturizing cream into your hair, make two braids, and go to bed (get some rest for less dark circles under your eyes). When you undo your braids in the morning, you'll have messy beach-y waves.

Hack 2: Multitask

Don't just do one thing at a time. There are plenty of beauty tasks you can do at the same time as your other morning tasks. You can brush your teeth as your hair conditioner soaks in, blow dry your hair while you catch up on email, or put on your make up while you wait for your coffee to brew.

Hack 3: Scarves

Another very easy way to glam up unwashed hair is to tie a scarf on. The Dolphin Fin tie, for instance, can be done in three step: fold the scarf, wrap it around your head, and tie a double knot, leaving the ends out. You'll look fun and polished without the hassle.

Hack 4: The Right Cut

Similar to splurging on a few trendy pieces of clothing to upgrade your wardrobe, hair can be splurged on as well. If you invest in a high quality cut, you'll reduce the time it takes to tame your mane in the morning. Go for something with a unique shape, like an asymmetrical bob, or something with layers. Your hair will stand out on its own without the tools and products.

Hack 5: Curl 'n' Go

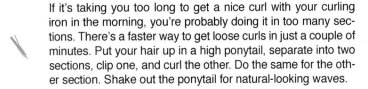

If it's taking you too long to get a nice curl with your curling iron in the morning, you're probably doing it in too many sections. There's a faster way to get loose curls in just a couple of minutes. Put your hair up in a high ponytail, separate into two sections, clip one, and curl the other. Do the same for the other section. Shake out the ponytail for natural-looking waves.

Tip! For thicker hair, use four sections instead of two.

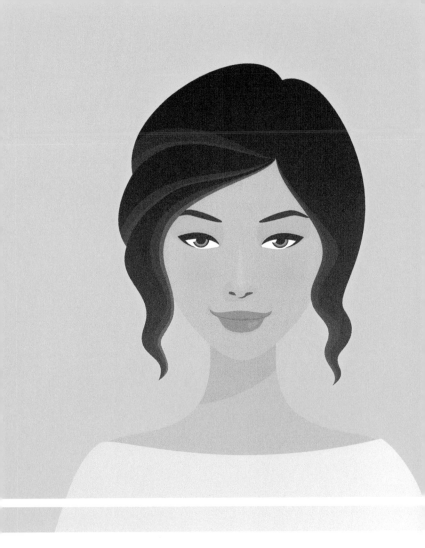

Hair //
Dirty Hair Tricks

It's not gross to skip a wash, everyone does it. Life gets busy. Luckily, there are plenty of ways to hide your dirty hair and look professional as heck.

Hack 1: Bang Wash

Want to skip shampooing but don't want stringy bangs? Wash them! Pull all of your hair back in a ponytail or with a clip, then wash your bangs. Make sure to use a proportional amount of shampoo and conditioner. Rinse under the faucet and blow dry if you don't have straight hair. Style your bangs as usual or use them to frame your face in a cute up-do.

Hack 2: Hat Trick

No time to wash your hair and out of dry shampoo (or baby powder)? Muss up your hair and put a hat on it. Done!

Hack 3: Skip a Wash

There's plenty of dry shampoo products on the market these days. If you put too much dry shampoo in your hair, just blow-dry it a little bit. Also, once you've massaged it into your hair, don't touch your hair! Your fingers will make it greasy. A bristle brush is better with dry shampoo and helps work the formula in more. And don't waste your dry shampoo – only spray it onto roots!

Tip! One thing to remember when applying dry shampoo is that you should let it sit in your hair untouched for 5-10 minutes before you massage it in. Let it really soak up the grease.

Hack 4: Quick Slick

Use that excess oil to your advantage by doing a quick, slick ponytail or bun. Brush hair through and shake out with a towel to get rid of any bed fuzz or dandruff. Flat iron any kinks. Next, use a hair gel or firm hold hair spray to slick hair back. Use an elastic to make a ponytail and take a small section of hair to wrap around the elastic and secure with a bobby pin for an extra chic look.

Hack 5: Instant Volume

 Use Velcro rollers at the crown of your head to instantly add volume to second or third day hair. Let the rollers sit while you brush your teeth and get dressed for work. By the time you take them off, it'll look like you just gave yourself a semi-fresh blowout!

Hack 6: Switch Sides

 In order to get a cleaner look, part your hair to the opposite site you usually do. Your hair will look cleaner and more voluminous. Spritz on some dry shampoo and run your fingers through the product to get some lift at the roots.

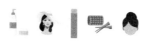

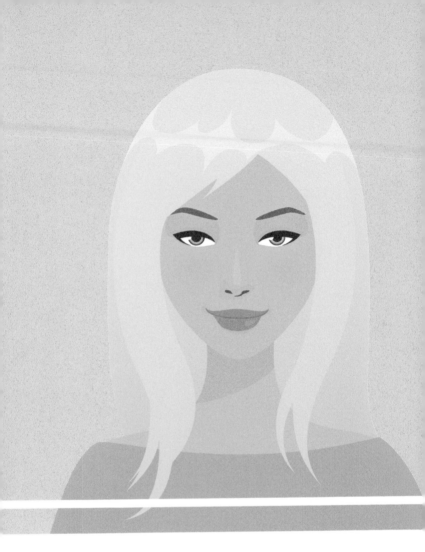

Hair //
Better Hair

Sometimes a little hack is all you need to fix up any style for your morning hair. Check out these fast tricks for making your hair look thicker and more polished in just minutes.

Hack 1: Instant Thick Hair

To make your hair look instantly thicker, brush a little eyeshadow on the middle of your part. Make sure the color matches your own hair color, and blend it well with your brush.

Hack 2: Clean Hairdryer

Use a toothbrush to clean the back end of your hairdryer. It'll last you longer and work better when you need it to.

Hack 3: Flyaways

Tame annoying flyaways with a little bit of hairspray on an old toothbrush. Spray on the hairspray and brush gently with the tooth brush. It'll catch the hairs that your bigger brush can't.

Hack 4: Hold It In

If you don't want to bother with fixing and re-fixing your hair all day long, spray your bobby pins with hairspray before you put them in. They'll hold your style much better than without the spray.

Hack 5: Fast Dry

Drying your hair takes so much work. Get a hair dryer holder and make your life a thousand times easier. Save so much time by drying your hair with a tee shirt instead of a towel.

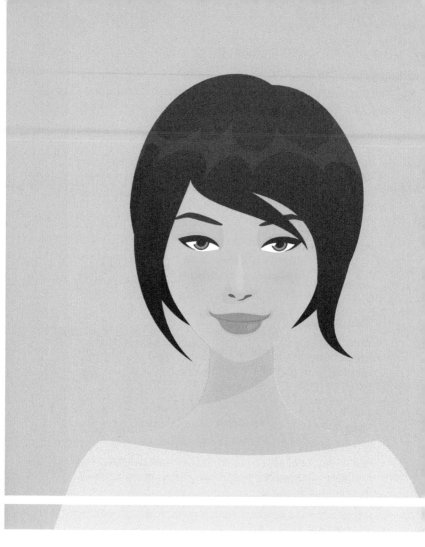

Hair //
Fast Styles

Here are some more looks to look professional before you head out the door. With a chic up do or a power ponytail, you'll worry less about your hair and more about your pressing work matters or a hot date.

Hack 1: Criss-Cross

This woven design immediately upgrades the classic second-day style to red carpet-worthy levels. First, gather up a ponytail, but separate a section of hair on each side and leave it loose. Next, separate each side into a top layer and a bottom layer. Cross each section over to the opposite side and pin in place.

Hack 2: Quick Updo

The Ballerina Bun is one of these incredibly simple buns that work almost anywhere. Simply pull your hair back into a ponytail so that it is sleek and free of bumps, then twist into a bun—and that's it.

Hack 3: Sleek Power Ponytail

Look polished in less than five minutes by pulling your hair up into a power ponytail, which is basically just an elevated version of your standard sporty pony. The secret? Wrapping your hair around your elastic for that extra chic factor.

Hack 4: Upside-Down Half Bun

An upgraded version of the basic half-up ponytail, the upside-down half bun is just as easy, but twice as chic. Just loop the tail of your pony into a bun, and no one will suspect you did your hair while waiting at a red light.

Hack 5: Messy Low Bun

With this style, dirty hair is encouraged. Haven't brushed your hair since Saturday (no judgment)? Muss it up even more and give yourself the messiest of messy low buns. Tie or pin it back.

Hack 6: Bobby Pin Art

Pull some hair back, secure it with bobby pins in the shape of a triangle or a crisscross design, and you're done! People will think you labored over the design, but it will only take you a minute or two.

Hack 7: Barely a Braid

Make a couple loops, tie it off, and go. It's an easy style, even for the amateur braider.

Hack 8: Low Pony

The low pony is the ultimate fast hairstyle. To give yours a little something extra, pull the pony tight, and then lift a few pieces right above the hair tie. This adds a bit of volume, ensuring you'll look a bit better than if you just rolled out of bed.

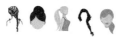

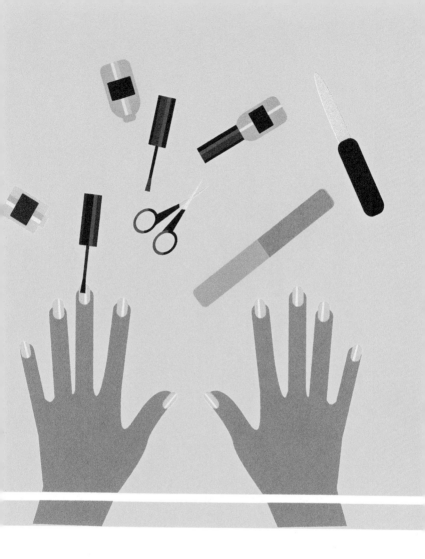

CHAPTER 4 //
Nails

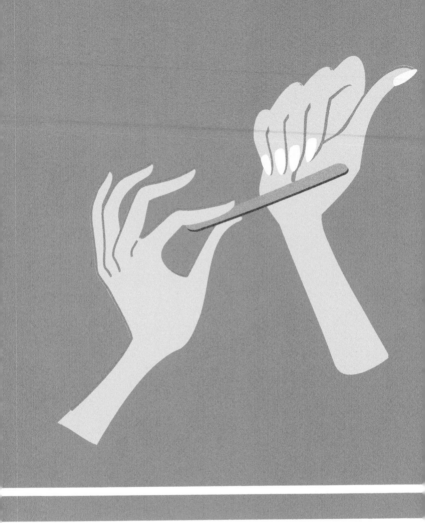

Nails //
Last-Minute Manicure

Nails seem like a high maintenance thing to pull off in the morning, but we've got your covered. There are plenty of ways to make your hands look polished and lovely before you run out the door. Here are some creative solutions for less mess with polish and more glam.

Hack 1: Gold Foil

If you wake up to find a can't-miss invitation for a special event sitting in your inbox, we've got you covered on the nail front. This festive gold-foil manicure is easy: get a dark nail color, a base coat, gold foil, and a topcoat. Swipe your nails with the base color and base coat, then use tweezers to place the bits of foil on your nails while the base coat is still wet, and use the topcoat to seal them in.

Hack 2: Fake Manicure

If your mornings are so hectic that your breakfast consists of two bites of whatever leftovers from the night before, then chances are you don't have time for a manicure. But that doesn't mean you have to step out into the world with dull nails. Instead of putting on a coat of color, quickly buff your nails for shine, and swipe on a clear nail strengthener for that polished look without the mess. Try buying an all-in-one top-coat, base coat, and strengthener for an even easier quickie manicure.

Hack 3: Whiten Those Nails

Sometimes you need to get the polish off, and you'd rather not have the big mess that comes along with it. There's no reason to look like you just competed in a finger-painting contest or soaked your nails in beer. Remove your polish. Then, soak your nails in a solution of hot water, hydrogen peroxide, and baking soda for about a minute.

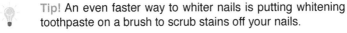

Tip! An even faster way to whiter nails is putting whitening toothpaste on a brush to scrub stains off your nails.

Hack 4: Know Your Colors

A quick way to know what your nail colors look like is to paint a small dot with a toothpick on the lid of each one, then place them in a container. If you need to whip up a manicure in minutes, it'll be easier to know which color to choose.

Hack 5: Fix a Smudge

If you accidentally smudge your nails while they're still wet, you can easily fix it by licking your finger and gently smoothing it out. You can also use your tongue to smoothen. It sounds gross, but your saliva reacts with the nail polish to soften and blend the surface and get back where it's supposed to go.

Hack 6: Polish Removal

If removing a dark nail polish tends to end up looking like you just did some gardening, here's a simple trick: apply a thick layer of hand cream before removing it. And try to apply pressure only on the nail when removing polish, then sliding the polish off, rather than spreading it all over your finger.

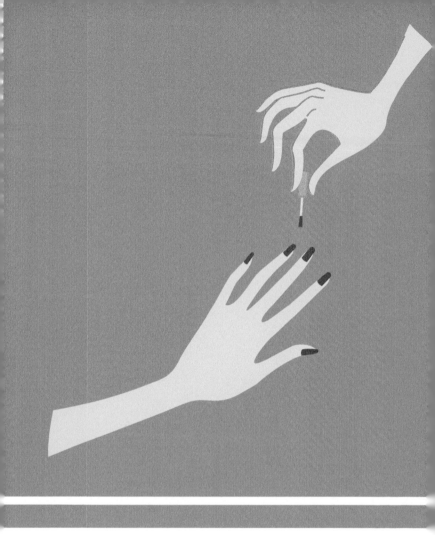

Nails //
Making Manicures Last

You've got your nails done, but oops! There they go getting chipped. Now you look like a little kid who's been running around playing with mom's beauty supplies. Fear not, we've got a few tricks up our sleeve to make that manicure last longer than just a day.

Hack 1: Perfect Gel

Gel polishes tend to last longer than regular nail polish, so they can be a good investment if you're not looking to do your nails every few days. Buy a good-quality gel polish kit. Apply base coat, then polish. Apply several coats of polish. If needed, let the nails settle under a UV lamp, but if you want to skip this step, make sure to buy a polish that doesn't require light to dry.

Hack 2: Vinegar Trick

Wipe down your nails with white vinegar and a cotton swab before applying basecoat. You'll remove any product buildup or natural oils on your nail beds. These would have created a barrier between the polish and your nail, but no more. Once your nails are dry, apply basecoat.

Hack 3: Don't Soak

Don't soak nails before painting them. Manicurists do this to soften cuticles, but it causes nails to retain water and expand. Once they're painted they'll shrink, meaning your polish will no longer fit your nails. So ask your manicurist to use cuticle oil instead.

Hack 4: Mirror Your Cuticle

File your nails into a shape that mirrors your cuticle's, which makes them less likely to break. And they'll look nice, too!

Hack 5: Avoid the Cuticle

Getting polish on your cuticles will lift the paint from the nail and lead to chipping, so avoid it. Don't cut your cuticles, as that could lead to infections, but you can push them back using cuticle oil and a pusher tools to prevent paint from getting on them.

Hack 6: Double Up

Apply two coats of basecoat to the tips of your nails. Nail tips are more prone to chipping (see: typing, texting, etc.). Apply another layer of basecoat to the top half of your nails for extra polish resilience.

Tip! Use a sticky base coat for extra protection.

Hack 7: Roll It

Roll your nail polish between your hands instead of shaking it up and down to get rid of air bubbles. You want to prevent bubbles, as painting them onto your nails will make them chip faster.

Hack 8: Cool Air

Dry nails with cool air. Hot air keep the polish from drying so use your blow dryer on its cool setting or a fan. Dipping fingertips in ice water for a minute or two also aids drying.

Hack 9: Skip the Sanitizer

Hand sanitizer dries out your nails and ruins topcoat, so cut it out of your cleaning routine. Wash your hands with mild soap instead, and preserve those nails.

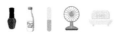

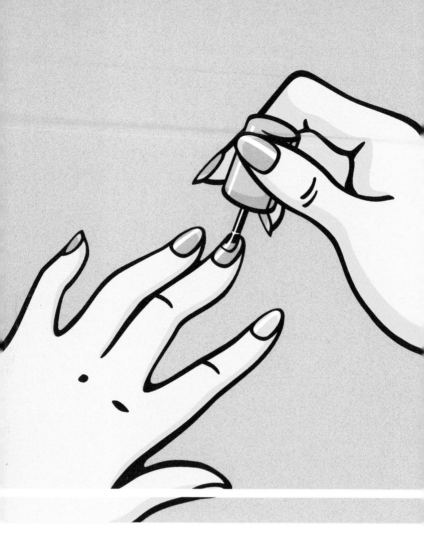

Nails //
Nail Techniques

Maintaining your nails doesn't have to be a hassle either. And you don't need a cabinet full of expensive products or frequent visits to the salon. All you need are a few household items and a little ingenuity from us.

Hack 1: Ice It

Use a bowl of ice water to dry your nails in three minutes, but let them air dry for a few minutes first.

Hack 2: Teabag and Glue

A broken nail can be fixed in a pinch with a piece of a teabag. Cut a tiny piece of the bag and place it under the broken part of the nail. Use nail glue to seal the deal.

Hack 3: Clean up Mistakes

Grab some skin cream on a Q-tip and put it around a nail that you've painted messily. Then wipe the stray paint off with a wooden nail tool.

Hack 4: Protect Your Hands

If you've ever had the displeasure of a split fingernail, you understand why it's important to protect your hands. Wear rubber or latex gloves while washing dishes or hand washing clothes to keep your manicure in tip-top shape and prevent cracked nails.

Hack 5: Restore Cuticles Overnight

Soak your fingers for 5 minutes in warm water. Then, push back your cuticles using an orange stick. Mix 3 tablespoons of lotion and 1 tablespoon of olive oil. Rub the mixture on your cuticles and nail beds.

Hack 6: Homemade Hand Scrub

If your hands have a lot of dead skin, lotion alone won't be able to soothe it. Consider creating hand scrub at home that has the same beneficial effects as the expensive stuff sold in stores. A blend of lemon, sugar, coconut oil, and Argan oil is instantly enriching while exfoliating skin.

Hack 7: Dry with Spray

With cooking spray or hair spray, you can dry your nails in a fast, cheap way. Spray a bit over the topcoat to strengthen the top layer and make it more resistant to smudges. It won't prevent major damage from occurring, however.

Hack 8: Repair Chipped Nails

Quickly cover up chips in nail polish with a coat of glitter. Choose a uniform pattern or apply glitter polish in varying strengths to achieve a faded effect.

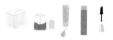

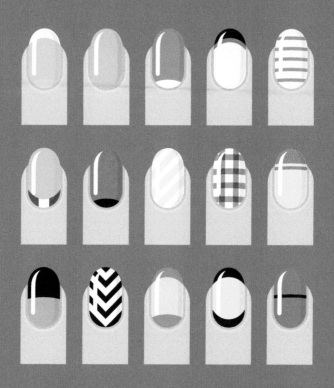

Nails //
Fast Nail Designs

Y ou're a little jealous of your friend's super cool manicure that she paid a fortune for at the salon. Forget all that—you can be a nail artist right at home and in no time at all.

Hack 1: DIY Glitter

Turn any clear nail polish into glitter polish by mixing it with craft glitter or eye shadow.

Hack 2: Sponge Paint Nails

Achieve a designer look with this spotted hack. Crumple up a plastic bag and dip in nail polish before using it to create a sponge paint effect on your nails. Press the bag onto your nails. Remember to use Vaseline on your skin to avoid spreading polish everywhere.

TIP! For best results, use a color that contrasts with the base coat.

Hack 3: Nail Tape

Nail tape is a great tool to keep around, whether you want to apply it directly to your nails or use it as a stencil for designs. To achieve perfectly straight lines, add it to your nail tips before applying the tip color.

Hack 4: I <3 It

Create a heart with a toothpick by placing two small dots next to each other on your nail. Then, create a "V" shape starting from those dots. With a little practice, you should be able to make adorable nail hearts in no time.

Hack 5: Gradient Nails

Create an interesting optical illusion is using gradients of color on your nails. This design is achieved by slightly blending two polish colors side by side, then using a sponge to apply the color to the nail.

Hack 6: Cutouts

Back to the nail tape! Apply strips of tape to the nail before polishing where you don't want the paint to land. Make cool geometric shapes with it. Use varying colors on each triangle before peeling tape off. You'll get a modern manicure worthy of your favorite sci-fi film.

Hack 7: Flowers

Get in the mood for springtime with easy floral nails. Simply make dots using a bobby pin or toothpick, then layer colors over the dots to create depth and the appearance of a flower. Add green accents to mimic leaves.

Hack 8: Matte Nails

Mix cornstarch with nail polish to get a matte topcoat you can use on any color. Paint your nails as you usually do, then add the topcoat!

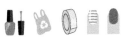

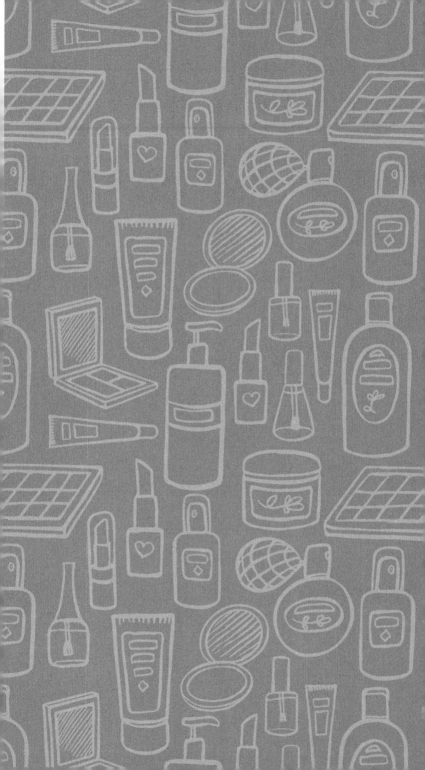

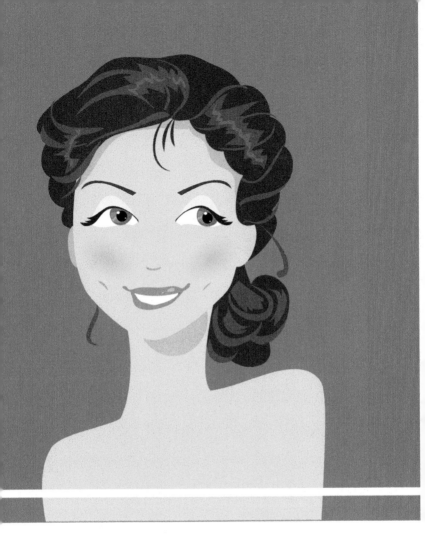

CHAPTER 5 //
Complete Morning Looks

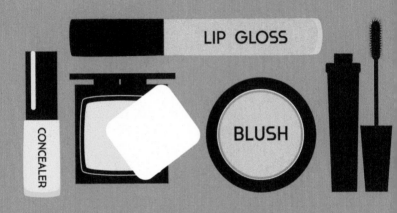

**Complete Morning Looks //
2-Minute Make-up**

If you've only got two minutes before you miss your bus or you'll show up late to work, we've got a method for you to get out the door in time.

Step 1: Use Ctoncealer

Use a brush to apply or your fingers. Apply to any blemishes that you want to cover up.

Step 2: Powder

Grab your powder and dust all over the face. It's great for absorbing excess oils. Make sure to apply to the neck as well.

Step 3: Blush

Apply with a brush on your cheeks.

Step 4: Mascara and Lip Gloss

Apply of bit of both of these, and you're good to go!

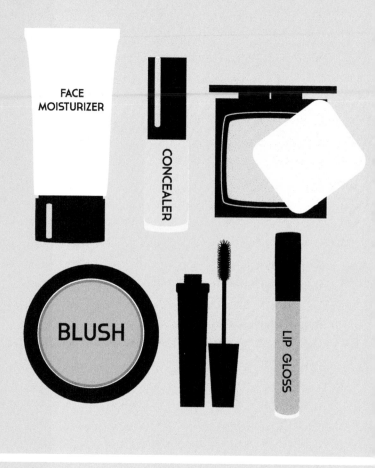

Complete Morning Looks //
3-Minute Everyday Look

Okay you've got one extra minute. Here's how to look like you didn't just roll out of bed.

Step 1: Tinted Moisturizer

Another option is to skip the foundation and use tinted moisturizer instead. Apply with your fingers. Dab all over your face, and make sure to blend evenly all over.

Step 2: Concealer

Grab a liquid concealer. Dot the concealer onto the bags and dark areas of your face.

Step 3: Pressed Powder

Brush on pressed powder. Swipe all over your face, but be sparing. The point is to dust it on, not cake it on.

Step 4: Apply Blush

Like in the last section, you'll be adding a little color to your face. Keep in mind that the most natural shade is the one that matches your face after you've been exercising or have been out in the cold.

Step 5: Grab the Mascara

Once again, you'll be opening up your eyes with mascara. Don't ditch it, as it makes a noticeable difference. Hold the mascara wand perpendicular to your eyelashes and start from the innermost part of your eyelashes. Keep most of the mascara at the base, to give the illusion of length

Step 6: Gloss

Swipe on some gloss, preferably with a natural pink tint, and run off to work!

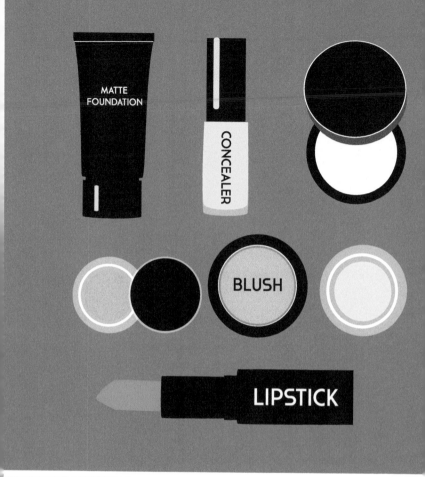

Complete Morning Looks //
5-Minute Natural Look

You've got a little more time, so let's give your face some more definition. Many of the steps are similar to the 2- and 3-minute looks, so if you're looking for something fast, go back to those.

Step 1: Foundation

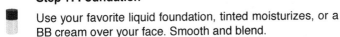

Use your favorite liquid foundation, tinted moisturizes, or a BB cream over your face. Smooth and blend.

Step 2: Concealer

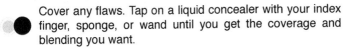

Cover any flaws. Tap on a liquid concealer with your index finger, sponge, or wand until you get the coverage and blending you want.

Step 3: Translucent Powder

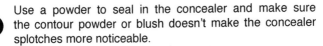

Use a powder to seal in the concealer and make sure the contour powder or blush doesn't make the concealer splotches more noticeable.

Step 4: Contour

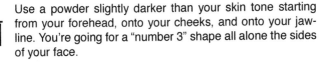

Use a powder slightly darker than your skin tone starting from your forehead, onto your cheeks, and onto your jaw-line. You're going for a "number 3" shape all alone the sides of your face.

Step 5: Blush

As usual, add blush!

Step 6: Highlight

Use a highlighter stick to highlight the bridge of your nose, the center of your forehead, your chin, the little dent above your upper lip, and just above your cheeks.

Step 7: Finishing Touches

Define your brows, throw on some mascara, and line and fill your lips with lipstick or lip gloss—but not all three if you don't have time. Remember what we said about mascara!

How to : **CONTOUR**

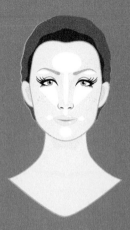

USE A FOUNDATION **2 SHADES LIGHTER** THAN YOUR SKIN TONE TO HIGHLIGHT.

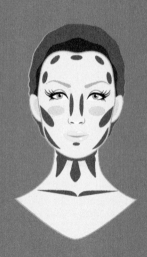

FOR CONTOURING USE A **LOW OR NON-SHIMMER** BRONZER. SET WITH POWDER.

HIGHLIGHT THE BRIDGE OF YOUR NOSE TO LIGHTEN THE FACE, AVOID THE TIP.

CONTOUR ON EACH SIDE OF THE NOSE TO MAKE IT LOOK MORE SLIM AND DEFINED.

CONTOUR AROUND THE HAIRLINE TO WARM THE FACE AND SHORTEN THE FOREHEAD.

CONTOUR ONE INCH ABOVE THE TEMPLE TO ADD DEPTH TO THE FACE.

HIGHLIGHT BETWEEN THE BROWS WHERE A FURROW MAY APPEAR.

CONTOUR THE UNDERSIDE OF THE CHEEKBONE TO STRENGTHEN YOUR BONE STRUCTURE.

HIGHLIGHT UNDER THE EYEBROW ARCH TO LIFE THE BROW AND BRIGHTEN THE EYES.

HIGHLIGHT THE HIGH POINT OF THE CHEKBONE TO DEFINE THE CHEEK.

CONTOUR THE TIP OF THE NOSE IN A V SHAPE TO SHORTEN THE LENGTH.

HIGHLIGHT CREASES THAT CREATE SHADOWS SUCH AS IN THE NASAL FOLD AREA.

CONTOUR UNDER THE JAW LINE TO ADD DEFINITION AND SLIM THE FACE.

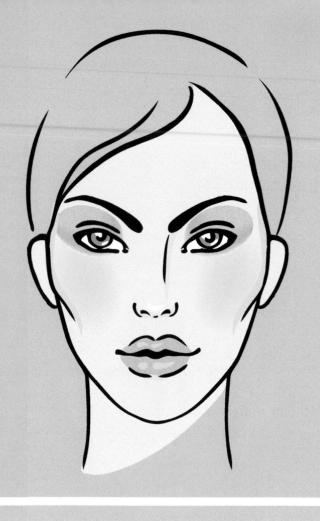

**Complete Morning Looks //
5-Minutes, 5 Products**

We're all about simplifying your routine, so why not get some fashionista looks into your repertoire? These are tried and true looks with as few products as possible—the magic number "3." They're recipes for glam!

Look 1: Watercolor Effect

A subtle sexy look that easily transitions from day to night: dab on a buildable gel eye shadow in a plum shade onto the lids with a brush or fingers. Then, blend out into the crease for a sheer wash color. Apply a peach lip and cheek stain first on the apples of your cheeks to get a sheer glossy look, then add a touch on the lips for a just-bitten effect. Finish the look off with black mascara; one coat is all you need.

Look 2: Pop of Red

A classic red lip is great all year round, but during the summer months it works best when you down play your other features. Pair your go-to crimson lipstick with a soft pink blush to balance out the pop of bold color and finish off with a few extra swipes of mascara to create a false lash effect.

Look 3: Bronze Glow

Nothing looks more summer appropriate than glowing skin and coral eye shadow. To achieve the look, swipe a bronzer (the one we suggest works on all skin tones) across your forehead, into the hollows of the cheeks, over the bridge of your nose, and along your jawline. Don't forget your shoulders and décolleté if you're showing some skin. To perfectly complement your bronzed glow, swipe a soft coral eye shadow gently across your lids and a clear lip balm on your lips.

Look 4: Bold Brow, Nude Lip

This sophisticated look has been going strong on the runway for the past few seasons, but can easily translate to real life. Create a well-groomed and defined brow by filling them in with a powder and setting with a pomade. Add one or two swipes of mascara—curl your lashes first and your eyes will seem brighter and more refreshed. Choose a nude lip that suits your skin tone to finish things off.

Look 5: Colorful Cat Eye

Choose a teal green eyeliner and draw along the upper lash winging up and out at the end to create a cat eye effect. Then apply two coats of mascara and complete the look with a lip gloss in a sheer, rose shade.

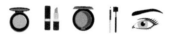

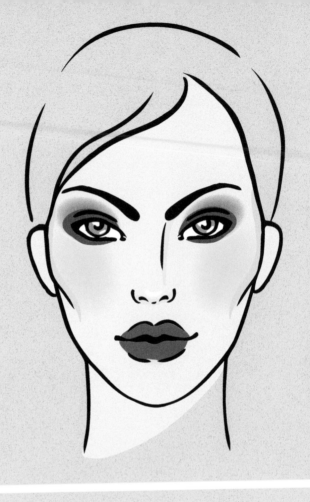

Complete Morning Looks //
10-Minutes to Glam

You've got 10 whole minutes! Let's really make them count with a sure-fire look that'll leave your co-workers stunned at how polished you seem every morning. It'll look like it took an hour, but we know it didn't, and that's a good thing.

Step 1: Prep

Like before, put on BB cream or foundation on your face. To save time, let it dry while you work on your eyes.

Step 2: Eyes

Start with an eye primer, usually in nude. Apply it with your fingers to hide all those visible blood vessels. Next, grab a shimmery neutral shade and apply in a light wash over the entire lid. Line your eyes with brown liner. Finish up with mascara, and curl your eyelashes if you'd like.

Step 3: Brows

You can skip this if you're pressed for time, but it'll add more definition to your face. Use a brow pencil to fill in your brows. It shouldn't take more than a minute.

Step 4: Face

Apply concealer in a triangle shape under your eyes, around your nostrils, and on any other imperfections that bug you. Next, set with powder. Apply blush either before or after the powder, depending on what you prefer. Applying powder after will tone down the shade of the blush a bit.

Step 5: Lips

The easiest way to maintain your lips all day is to use a tinted lip balm. It won't fade or get on your teeth the way lipstick does, and it's very easy to re-apply.

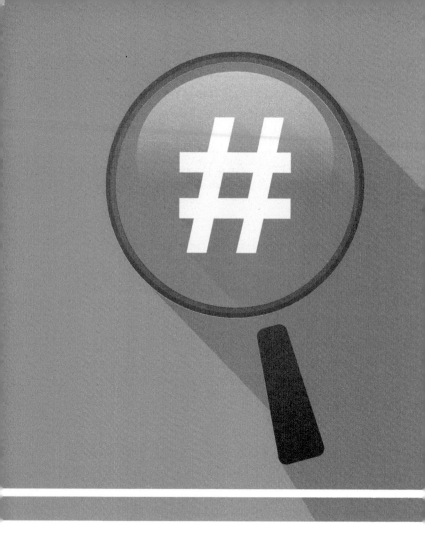

**Complete Morning Looks //
#trendingtips**

Wigs US @WigsUS Using eye creams help smooth the fine lines and crow's feet and prevent premature aging around the eyes. #BeautyTips

Naturals @Naturals3000 Curl your eyelashes twice before you apply #mascara to create a more youthful look. #BeautyTips

ULearn Beauty @ULearn_Beauty Use a flesh colored liner on the water rim of your lower lash line to make eyes look bigger and brighter #beautytips

Diva Likes @Diva_Likes Beware of brown eye shadow shades that are reddish, as they can make you look tired or (worse) hungover #beautytips

RAW Pressery @RawPressery Skip bubble bath & salts, & add coconut oil to your bath. Hot water will melt the oil into a liquid & leave you #moisturized. #BeautyTips

CaroLina Beauty @CaroLina_Beauty The most important rule when wearing a smoky eye is that if you go dark, keep the rest of your face soft #beautytips

Manila Barbie @manilabarbie Change out your mascara every three months When it comes to your eyes, it's better to be safe than sorry #beautytips

Agustina Beauty Tips @agustinawzb23 Use a primer on your eyebrows before applying pencil or powder It'll make the product stay on much longer #beautytips

rmsyplt @clkbnk If you're constantly waking up to puffy #eyes, consider changing your laundry detergent You may be allergic #beautytips

Lorion Beauty @LorionBeauty Brushes hold #foundation better than fingers, meaning you can spread it thinly for a more #natural look. #beautytips

Classic Beauty @ClassicBeauty If your lashes are already clumped, take a spiral brush and remove the mascara by swirling against the lashes #beautytips

Camp Hopson @CampHopson Don't touch your face unless you have to... spots can be caused from your own fingers and the bacteria they carry #QuickBeauty

per-fékt beauty @perfekt_beauty Use a drop-sized amount of cheek perfection gel. Smile & pat onto apple of cheeks, then smooth upwards. #easybeauty

The Body Shop India @TheBodyShopIND #BeautyTip - Reduce unwanted shine by using a moisturizer that mattifies your skin & provides the required moisture without making it greasy

Beauty at Tesco @BeautyatTesco Match your lip liner to your own lip colour rather than your lipstick for a natural outline. #beautytip

Glam and Glitter @GlamandGlitter Give your hair a blast with cool air to help 'set' your style & prevent it drooping as it cools gradually.#beautytip

Trufora @Trufora Toss chia seeds into your smoothie - they're rich in fatty acids that erase blemishes, soften wrinkles & help keep skin hydrated! #beautytip brodieandstone @brodieandstone Keep your nail polishes in the fridge - they'll glide on smoother and last longer without chips! #BeautyTip

Latest in Beauty @LatestInBeauty #BeautyTip to minimise old acne scars, start introducing a peptide based peel into your skincare regime. It works wonders!

Beauty Resource @BeautyResource #BeautyTip: Use a touch of highlighter on your cupids bow to emphasise your lips.

FACE atelier @FACEatelier Wiggle your #mascara brush in little left-right motions as you apply. It reduces clumps and gives a more even application. #BeautyTip

Preen.Me @preendotme Boost your #confidence when you maintain proper #posture at all times. It makes one look really good! #BeautyTip

the diviners @The_Diviners Have you tried putting on a face mask with a brush? Because it's the best thing ever. #beauty #pamper

Beaute La Royale @beautelaroyale Want baby soft skin? Mix avocado and honey, apply it to your face for 15 minutes then rinse! #SkinCare #BeautyTip

Beauty Image USA @BeautyImageUSA Use foundation, not concealer (which is lighter than your #skin color), to cover up redness or blemishes. #looking-good

Natural World @naturalworld_ #BeautyTips Dip dyed your hair? Always use a nourishing hair mask conditioner and concentrate on your dyed ends!

Beauty Resource @BeautyResource #BeautyTip: Don't pump your mascara wand - this gets air into the container and dries out the product.

Pretty Dollfaced AZ @PrettyDollfaced Hot showers dry out your #skin. When you turn red & itchy, it's time to step out! #BeautyTip

A NOTE FROM THE AUTHORS

Beauty is an ill-defined term for looking healthy, pleasant, or sexy, but really we just want you to feel like yourself. A put-together version of yourself that gets to sleep 20 extra minutes every morning and still looks good walking out the door. What's looking good? It's up to you really. However you want to smear these weird concoctions on your face is your choice. Or if you don't want to use any at all—that's cool too. We hope you like our hacks and tweet some to us (**#BeautyHacks**) at **@mangomediainc**. Good luck on all your make up or make up-less adventures!

DATA SOURCES

http://stylecaster.com/beauty-high/beauty-uses-for-household-items/

https://www.pinterest.com/pin/293226625714295373/

https://www.pinterest.com/pin/379920918541721260/

https://www.pinterest.com/pin/AZHha9J5k_mqPgHatJeLyxfXHEf45tWNiyi4p8lsxPSWcixEy9hFiGY/

https://www.pinterest.com/pin/168322104794369262/

https://www.pinterest.com/pin/141581982011019385/

https://www.pinterest.com/pin/174514554287263087/

https://www.pinterest.com/pin/108227197270243358/

https://www.pinterest.com/pin/130252614199437337/

https://www.pinterest.com/pin/422212533788745265/

OTHER SOURCES

http://www.goodhousekeeping.com/beauty/anti-aging/tips/a27077/overnight-skin-tips/

http://www.popsugar.com/beauty/Beauty-Tips-Save-Time-Morning-36523705#photo-undefined

http://www.refinery29.com/how-to-look-awake

http://www.popsugar.com/beauty/Look-Awake-When-Youre-Tired-Olay-Fresh-Effects-36045068

http://www.dailymail.co.uk/femail/article-3106052/Use-red-lipstick-eyes-apply-concealer-triangle-shape-use-SPOONS-beat-bags-simple-beauty-hacks-cheat-8-hours-sleep.html

http://www.cosmopolitan.com/style-beauty/beauty/how-to/a34361/lipstick-hacks/

http://www.teen.com/2014/12/11/style/beauty-news-trends-ideas-celebrity-inspiration/eyebrow-hacks-tips-tricks-how-to-pictures/

http://www.diyncrafts.com/3312/fashion/40-diy-beauty-hacks-borderline-genius/5

http://www.whowhatwear.com/how-to-fill-in-your-eyebrows-like-a-pro

http://youqueen.com/beauty/hair/easy-updos/

http://www.gurl.com/2014/12/16/hacks-tips-and-tricks-how-to-use-dry-shampoo/

http://diply.com/different-solutions/23-hairstyle-hacks-lazy-girl-in-you/31440

http://www.cosmopolitan.com/style-beauty/beauty/advice/a33593/longer-lasting-manicure-tricks/

http://nails.allwomenstalk.com/awesome-nails-hacks-that-make-painting-your-nails-a-breeze/2/

http://www.lifehack.org/articles/lifestyle/every-girl-needs-these-30-nail-hacks-for-the-perfect-mani-cure.html

http://www.bouvardian.com/5-minute-face/

http://www.elle.com/beauty/makeup-skin-care/news/a25048/3-product-makeup-looks/

http://www.15minutebeauty.com/2015/02/my-current-makeup-routine.html?m=1

CPSIA information can be obtained at www.ICGtesting.com
Printed in the USA
BVOWf1s1933060116

431948BV00005B/6/P